THINK BIG AND WORK SMART

Journey Through A Healthier life

By

LILIAN W. JOHNSON

TABLE OF CONTENTS

- Understanding the difference between a fixed mindset and a growth mindset
- Why a growth mindset is important for weight loss success
- Strategies for developing a growth mindset

PART THREE

- Working Smart
- Nutrition Basics
- Understanding the role of nutrition in weight loss
- The fundamentals of healthy eating
- Strategies for creating a sustainable nutrition plan
- Exercise and Movement
- The benefits of exercise for weight loss
- Types of exercise and finding what works for you

INTRODUCTION

"Think Big and Work Smart in Your Weight Loss Journey" is a comprehensive guide to achieving successful and lasting weight loss. The book is written by an experienced weight loss coach who believes in the power of setting big goals and working smart to achieve them.

The author's approach to weight loss is focused on two key principles: thinking big and working smart. In the first part of the book, the author encourages readers to set big, achievable goals for their weight loss journey. She provides practical tips for goal-setting and offers advice on how to stay motivated throughout the process.

The second part of the book focuses on working smart to achieve weight loss goals. The author covers nutrition basics, exercise and movement, mindful eating and portion control, and overcoming obstacles. She emphasizes the importance of creating a sustainable nutrition plan, finding an exercise routine that works for you, and practicing mindful eating to overcome cravings and emotional eating.

Throughout the book, the author emphasizes the importance of developing a growth mindset and staying motivated even when faced with setbacks. She provides practical strategies for overcoming obstacles and building a support system for long-term success.

Overall, "Think Big and Work Smart in Your Weight Loss Journey" offers a practical and holistic approach to weight loss that emphasizes the power of mindset, goal-setting, and sustainable lifestyle changes. The book is an excellent resource for anyone looking to achieve lasting weight loss success.

IMPORTANCE OF SETTING BIG GOALS AND WORKING SMART

Setting big goals and working smart are both important factors in achieving success, including weight loss success. Here's why:

✓ Motivation: Setting big goals can help you stay motivated and focused on your weight loss journey. When you have a clear idea of what you want to achieve, you're more likely to stay committed and put in the effort required to reach your goal.

✓ Direction: Big goals provide direction for your weight loss journey. They help you identify what you need to do in order to achieve your desired outcome, and guide your decision-making process.

✓ Progress: Working smart helps you make progress towards your goals more efficiently. By focusing on the strategies and techniques that are most effective, you can make progress faster and avoid wasting time on ineffective methods.

✓ Sustainability: Working smart also helps you create sustainable lifestyle changes that support long-term weight loss success. By identifying the habits and behaviors that are most effective for you, you can create a plan that is both effective and sustainable.

Overall, setting big goals and working smart are important because they provide motivation, direction, and efficiency in achieving weight loss success. By combining these two factors, you can create a clear plan for your weight loss journey that is both effective and sustainable.

PART ONE

GOAL-SETTING FOR WEIGHT LOSS

Goal-setting is a critical component of weight loss success. It involves creating specific, measurable, achievable, relevant, and time-bound (SMART) goals that provide direction and motivation for your weight loss journey. Here are some reasons why goal-setting is essential for weight loss:

Clarity: Setting specific goals can provide clarity about what you want to achieve and how to achieve it. This, in turn, can help you create a clear plan for your weight loss journey and guide your decision-making process.

Motivation: Goals provide motivation by giving you something to strive for. When you set goals that are important to you, you're more likely to stay committed and put in the effort required to achieve them.

Accountability: Setting goals can help you stay accountable to yourself and others. By sharing your goals with friends, family, or a weight loss coach, you're more likely to stick to them and make progress towards achieving them.

Progress: Goals provide a way to track your progress towards your weight loss goals. When you set specific, measurable goals, you can monitor your progress and make adjustments as needed to stay on track.

When setting weight loss goals, it's important to create goals that are realistic and achievable. Avoid setting goals that are too ambitious or unrealistic, as this can lead to frustration and disappointment. Instead, focus on creating goals that are challenging yet achievable, and that provide direction and motivation for your weight loss journey.

In summary, goal-setting is an essential component of weight loss success. By creating specific, measurable, achievable, relevant, and time-bound goals, you can create a clear plan for your weight loss journey, stay motivated, stay accountable, and track your progress towards achieving your desired outcome.

Why setting goals is important for weight loss success

Losing weight can be a challenging and often frustrating process. Many people struggle to achieve their weight loss goals despite their best efforts, leading to feelings of disappointment and defeat. However, setting goals is one of the most important steps you can take to achieve lasting weight loss success. Here are some reasons why setting goals is essential for weight loss:

Provides Direction: Setting specific goals provides direction for your weight loss journey. Goals help you identify what you want to achieve and provide a roadmap for how to get there. When you have a clear idea of where you're going, you're more likely to stay committed and motivated throughout the process.

Increases Motivation: Goals give you something to strive for, which can increase your motivation to succeed. When you have a clear goal in mind, you're more likely to put in the effort required to achieve it. Moreover, achieving your goals can be incredibly rewarding and can help you stay motivated to continue making progress towards your ultimate goal.

Builds Accountability: Setting goals can help build accountability. By sharing your goals with friends, family, or a weight loss coach, you're more likely to stay on track and make progress towards achieving your goals. When others know about your goals, you're more likely to stick to them and make the necessary changes to achieve success.

Allows for Measurable Progress: Goals provide a way to track your progress towards achieving your desired outcome. When you set specific, measurable goals, you can monitor your progress and make adjustments as needed to stay on track.

This can help you stay motivated and ensure that you're making steady progress towards your ultimate goal.

Creates a Sense of Control: Setting goals can help create a sense of control over your weight loss journey. When you have clear goals in mind, you can take ownership of your weight loss journey and make informed decisions about the steps you need to take to achieve success.

In conclusion, setting goals is an essential component of weight loss success. Goals provide direction, motivation, accountability, measurable progress, and a sense of control over your weight loss journey. By setting specific, achievable goals and staying committed to achieving them, you can achieve the body and health you've always wanted. Remember, the key is to set realistic goals that provide direction and motivation for your weight loss journey.

THE SMART METHOD FOR SETTING ACHIEVABLE GOALS

The SMART method is a popular goal-setting framework that helps individuals set achievable goals. SMART is an acronym for Specific, Measurable, Achievable, Relevant, and Time-bound. Here's a breakdown of each component:

Specific: Goals should be specific and clearly defined. This means avoiding vague or general goals and focusing on specific outcomes. For example, instead of setting a goal to "lose weight," you might set a goal to "lose 10 pounds in 2 months."

Measurable: Goals should be measurable so that you can track your progress and determine if you're making progress towards achieving your goal. Measurable goals often involve quantifiable outcomes, such as tracking the number of pounds lost or the number of calories consumed.

Achievable: Goals should be achievable, meaning they are realistic and within your reach. Setting goals that are too ambitious or unrealistic can lead to feelings of disappointment and defeat. Ensure that your goals are challenging yet attainable, given your current circumstances and resources.

Relevant: Goals should be relevant to your overall weight loss journey and aligned with your values and priorities. Ensure that your goals are meaningful and contribute to your overall well-being.

Time-bound: Goals should have a specific timeline or deadline for completion. This helps create urgency and motivation to achieve the goal within the designated time frame. For example, setting a goal to "lose 10 pounds in 2 months" is time-bound because it has a specific deadline for completion.

By using the SMART method, you can set achievable goals that provide direction and motivation for your weight loss journey. Remember, setting specific, measurable, achievable, relevant, and time-bound goals can help you stay on track and make steady progress towards achieving your desired outcome.

TIPS FOR STAYING MOTIVATED THROUGHOUT THE GOAL-SETTING PROCESS

Staying motivated throughout the goal-setting process is essential for achieving success in your weight loss journey. Here are some tips for staying motivated and on track towards your goals:

Keep your goals in mind: Keep your goals in mind by writing them down and posting them somewhere visible. This can serve as a daily reminder of what you're working towards and help you stay focused on your goals.

Celebrate small victories: Celebrate small victories along the way. Recognize and reward

yourself for making progress towards your goals.
This can help you stay motivated and reinforce
positive behaviors.

Find a support system: Find a support system of
friends, family, or a weight loss coach who can
provide encouragement and hold you
accountable. Having a support system can help
you stay motivated and make progress towards
your goals.

Track your progress: Keep track of your
progress towards your goals. This can help you
see the progress you've made and identify areas
where you need to make improvements.

Mix things up: Mix things up by trying new
exercises or healthy recipes. Keeping things
fresh and interesting can help prevent boredom
and maintain motivation.

Stay positive: Stay positive and focus on the
progress you're making, rather than setbacks or
mistakes. Recognize that setbacks are a natural

part of the process and use them as an opportunity to learn and grow.

Visualize success: Visualize yourself achieving your goals and imagine how it will feel to reach your desired outcome. This can help motivate you to stay committed to your goals.

In conclusion, staying motivated throughout the goal-setting process is essential for achieving success in your weight loss journey. By keeping your goals in mind, celebrating small victories, finding a support system, tracking your progress, mixing things up, staying positive, and visualizing success, you can stay motivated and on track towards achieving your desired outcome. Remember, staying motivated requires effort and commitment, but the rewards of achieving your weight loss goals are worth it in the end.

PART TWO

INTRODUCTION TO VISUALIZATION TECHNIQUES

Visualization techniques are powerful tools that can help individuals achieve their goals by harnessing the power of the mind. Visualization involves creating a mental image or scenario of a desired outcome or goal, using all the senses to create a vivid and detailed picture in the mind. When used correctly, visualization techniques can help individuals overcome obstacles, boost their confidence, and achieve success in various areas of their lives, including weight loss.

The concept of visualization has been around for centuries and has been used in various fields, from sports psychology to business management. The power of visualization lies in its ability to stimulate the brain and create a mental blueprint of what we want to achieve, which can help us stay motivated, focused, and on track towards our goals.

In the context of weight loss, visualization techniques can help individuals create a mental picture of themselves at their desired weight, imagining the feeling of being healthy and confident. By visualizing success, individuals can stay motivated, overcome challenges, and make progress towards achieving their weight loss goals.

In this article, we will explore different visualization techniques that can help individuals achieve their weight loss goals, including guided imagery, affirmations, and vision boards. We will also discuss the benefits of visualization and how to incorporate visualization techniques into a weight loss program for maximum effectiveness.

THE POWER OF VISUALIZATION IN ACHIEVING WEIGHT LOSS GOALS

The power of visualization is a well-established concept that has been used in various fields, including sports psychology, business management, and personal development. When applied to weight loss, visualization techniques can be an effective tool for helping individuals achieve their weight loss goals.

Visualization involves creating a mental image of a desired outcome or goal, using all the senses to create a vivid and detailed picture in the mind. The process of visualization stimulates the brain and creates a mental blueprint of what we want to achieve, which can help us stay motivated, focused, and on track towards our goals.

Studies have shown that visualization techniques can be effective for weight loss. In one study, overweight women were asked to visualize themselves as healthy, fit, and active. The women who engaged in visualization techniques lost more weight than those who did not. Another study found that visualization techniques were effective in helping individuals reduce their cravings for unhealthy foods.

The benefits of visualization in weight loss go beyond just motivation and focus. Visualization can also help individuals overcome obstacles and challenges, boost their confidence, and improve their self-esteem. By creating a mental picture of success, individuals can train their minds to believe in their ability to achieve their weight loss goals, which can help them stay committed and persistent.

There are several visualization techniques that individuals can use to achieve their weight loss goals, including:

Guided Imagery: Guided imagery involves creating a mental picture of a specific scene or scenario that evokes positive emotions and feelings. For weight loss, this might involve visualizing yourself engaging in healthy activities, such as exercising or eating nutritious foods.

Affirmations: Affirmations involve repeating positive statements to yourself, such as "I am capable of achieving my weight loss goals" or "I am strong and committed to my health". Repeating these affirmations can help reprogram negative thought patterns and increase motivation.

Vision Boards: Vision boards involve creating a visual representation of your weight loss goals, such as a collage of images or words that represent your desired outcome. Looking at the vision board regularly can help keep your goals in mind and provide a source of inspiration and motivation.

In conclusion, the power of visualization is a valuable tool for achieving weight loss goals. By creating a mental picture of success, individuals can stay motivated, overcome obstacles, and make progress towards their goals. Incorporating visualization techniques into a weight loss program can help individuals achieve long-term success and lead a healthier, happier life.

Techniques for visualizing your desired outcome

Visualization techniques are a powerful tool that can help individuals achieve their desired outcomes by harnessing the power of the mind. In the context of weight loss, visualization involves creating a mental image of a desired outcome or goal, using all the senses to create a vivid and detailed picture in the mind. Here are some techniques for visualizing your desired weight loss outcome:

Create a Mental Picture: One of the most effective ways to visualize your desired outcome is to create a mental picture of what you want to achieve. Close your eyes and imagine yourself at your desired weight, feeling healthy, energetic, and confident. Use all of your senses to create a detailed mental image, including sights, sounds, and sensations.

Use Guided Imagery: Guided imagery involves using a recording or script to guide your visualization process. There are many guided imagery resources available online that are specifically tailored to weight loss. These resources can help you create a mental image of yourself at your desired weight and motivate you to achieve your goals.

Create a Vision Board: A vision board is a visual representation of your goals and aspirations. Create a collage of images, words, and phrases that represent your desired outcome. Display your vision board in a prominent location, such as your bedroom or office, and look at it often to reinforce your visualization process.

Use Positive Affirmations: Affirmations are positive statements that help reinforce your visualization process. Repeat positive affirmations to yourself, such as "I am capable of achieving my weight loss goals" or "I am healthy and fit." Repeat these affirmations often, both during your visualization process and throughout the day.

Practice Mindfulness: Mindfulness involves being present in the moment and focusing your attention on your thoughts and feelings. Practicing mindfulness can help you stay focused on your weight loss goals and reinforce your visualization process.

In conclusion, visualization techniques are a powerful tool for achieving weight loss goals. By creating a mental picture of your desired outcome, using guided imagery, creating a vision board, using positive affirmations, and practicing mindfulness, you can stay motivated, focused, and on track towards achieving your weight loss goals.

Incorporating visualization into your daily routine

Incorporating visualization into your daily routine can be a powerful way to reinforce your weight loss goals and help you stay motivated. Here are some tips for incorporating visualization into your daily routine:

Set aside dedicated visualization time: Find a time each day when you can dedicate a few minutes to visualization. This could be in the morning, before bed, or during a lunch break. Whatever time works best for you, make sure it is consistent and part of your daily routine.

Use a visualization journal: Keep a visualization journal where you can write down your goals, positive affirmations, and any insights or revelations that come to you during your visualization process. This can help you stay focused and reinforce your visualization process.

Incorporate visualization into exercise: Use your exercise routine as an opportunity to visualize your desired outcome. Picture yourself at your desired weight and feeling strong and healthy as you work out. This can help motivate you during your workouts and reinforce your visualization process.

Use visualization during meals: Before each meal, take a few moments to visualize yourself making healthy food choices and enjoying your meal in a relaxed and mindful way. This can help you make healthier food choices and reinforce your visualization process.

Create reminders: Use reminders throughout the day to help reinforce your visualization process. This could be a reminder on your phone or computer, a post-it note on your desk, or a visualization trigger such as a specific song or image.

In conclusion, incorporating visualization into your daily routine can be a powerful way to reinforce your weight loss goals and stay motivated. By setting aside dedicated visualization time, using a visualization journal, incorporating visualization into exercise and meals, and creating reminders, you can make visualization a natural part of your daily routine and achieve success in your weight loss journey.

Developing a Growth Mindset

Developing a growth mindset is a key element in achieving success in any area of life, including weight loss. A growth mindset is the belief that our abilities and intelligence can be developed and improved through hard work, dedication, and learning from our failures. This is in contrast to a fixed mindset, which is the belief that our abilities and intelligence are fixed traits that cannot be changed.

Here are some ways to develop a growth mindset in your weight loss journey:

Embrace challenges: Instead of shying away from challenges, embrace them as opportunities to learn and grow. See challenges as a chance to develop new skills, overcome obstacles, and become stronger.

Learn from your mistakes: Instead of seeing mistakes as failures, see them as opportunities to learn and improve. Identify what went wrong and what you can do differently next time.

Remember that every mistake is a chance to grow and develop.

Focus on effort and progress: Instead of focusing solely on the end result, focus on the effort and progress you are making towards your goals. Celebrate small victories and milestones along the way, and recognize that progress is a process.

Cultivate a love of learning: Instead of seeing weight loss as a chore, cultivate a love of learning about nutrition, exercise, and healthy habits. Read books and articles, watch documentaries, and experiment with new recipes and workouts.

Surround yourself with positivity: Surround yourself with positive people who believe in you and support your goals. Avoid negative self-talk and cultivate a positive and supportive inner dialogue.

In conclusion, developing a growth mindset is a crucial element in achieving success in weight loss. By embracing challenges, learning from mistakes, focusing on effort and progress, cultivating a love of learning, and surrounding yourself with positivity, you can develop the mindset necessary to achieve your weight loss goals and become the best version of yourself.

Understanding the difference between a fixed mindset and a growth mindset
The terms "fixed mindset" and "growth mindset" were coined by psychologist Carol Dweck to describe two different ways of thinking about intelligence, abilities, and talents. A fixed mindset is the belief that our abilities, intelligence, and talents are fixed traits that cannot be changed. In contrast, a growth mindset is the belief that our abilities, intelligence, and talents can be developed and improved through hard work, dedication, and learning from our failures.

Here are some key differences between a fixed mindset and a growth mindset:

Belief in the ability to improve: A fixed mindset is characterized by a belief that our abilities and intelligence are fixed traits that cannot be changed. A growth mindset, on the other hand, is characterized by a belief that our abilities and intelligence can be developed and improved through hard work, dedication, and learning from our failures.

Response to challenges: Those with a fixed mindset tend to avoid challenges, as they see them as a threat to their self-image. Those with a growth mindset, on the other hand, see challenges as opportunities to learn and grow.

Response to failure: Those with a fixed mindset tend to see failure as evidence of their lack of ability or intelligence, and may give up when faced with failure. Those with a growth mindset see failure as an opportunity to learn and improve, and may even become more motivated after a setback.

Focus on effort versus talent: Those with a fixed mindset tend to focus on their inherent talents and abilities, while those with a growth mindset focus on their effort and dedication. Those with a growth mindset believe that hard work and dedication can lead to success, even if they do not have innate talent.

Openness to feedback: Those with a fixed mindset tend to be defensive and resistant to feedback, as they see it as a threat to their self-image. Those with a growth mindset are open to feedback, as they see it as an opportunity to learn and improve.

In conclusion, understanding the difference between a fixed mindset and a growth mindset is important in all areas of life, including weight loss. By cultivating a growth mindset and embracing challenges, learning from mistakes, focusing on effort and progress, and surrounding yourself with positivity, you can develop the mindset necessary to achieve your weight loss goals and become the best version of yourself.

Why a growth mindset is important for weight loss success

A growth mindset is important for weight loss success because it allows you to approach the journey with a positive and proactive attitude. When you have a growth mindset, you believe that you can develop the skills and habits necessary to achieve your goals, and that setbacks and failures are opportunities to learn and grow.

Here are some specific reasons why a growth mindset is important for weight loss success:

Resilience: A growth mindset allows you to bounce back from setbacks and failures more easily. When you encounter a challenge or obstacle on your weight loss journey, you are more likely to see it as an opportunity to learn and grow, rather than a sign of your inherent limitations.

Willingness to take risks: When you have a growth mindset, you are more willing to take risks and try new things. This can be important in weight loss, as you may need to experiment with different diets, exercise routines, and lifestyle changes to find what works best for you.

Focus on progress: A growth mindset helps you focus on progress and improvement, rather than perfection. Instead of getting discouraged by slow progress or small setbacks, you can celebrate the small wins and focus on the positive changes you are making.

Long-term perspective: A growth mindset encourages you to think about the long-term rather than the short-term. Instead of trying to lose weight quickly, you can focus on developing sustainable habits and making lasting changes that will help you maintain a healthy weight over time.

In conclusion, a growth mindset is an essential ingredient for weight loss success. By embracing challenges, learning from mistakes, focusing on progress, and believing in your ability to improve, you can develop the resilience, flexibility, and long-term perspective necessary to achieve your weight loss goals and maintain a healthy lifestyle over the long-term.

Strategies for developing a growth mindset
Developing a growth mindset can be challenging, especially if you have been stuck in a fixed mindset for a long time. However, with practice and persistence, you can shift your mindset and develop a more positive and proactive approach to weight loss. Here are some strategies for developing a growth mindset:

Embrace challenges: Instead of avoiding challenges or feeling overwhelmed by them, try to embrace them as opportunities to learn and grow. When you encounter a challenge or obstacle on your weight loss journey, ask yourself, "What can I learn from this?" or "How can I use this experience to become a better version of myself?"

Focus on effort and progress: Instead of focusing solely on outcomes, try to focus on the effort and progress you are making. Celebrate small wins and milestones along the way, and don't get discouraged by slow progress or setbacks.

Learn from mistakes: Instead of seeing mistakes as failures, try to view them as opportunities to learn and improve. When you make a mistake or experience a setback, ask yourself, "What can I learn from this?" or "What can I do differently next time?"

Adopt a growth mindset language: The words you use can have a powerful impact on your mindset. Instead of using language that reinforces a fixed mindset (e.g. "I'm not good at this," "I'll never be able to do it"), try to use language that reinforces a growth mindset (e.g.

"I can improve with practice," "I'm willing to try new things").

Surround yourself with growth-minded people: Surrounding yourself with people who have a growth mindset can be incredibly helpful in shifting your own mindset. Seek out friends, family members, or support groups who are positive, supportive, and focused on growth and improvement.

By incorporating these strategies into your daily life, you can gradually shift your mindset from a fixed mindset to a growth mindset, and develop the resilience, flexibility, and positive attitude necessary to achieve your weight loss goals and maintain a healthy lifestyle over the long-term.

PART THREE

NUTRITION BASICS

Nutrition is a fundamental aspect of weight loss and overall health. To achieve your weight loss goals, it's essential to understand the basics of nutrition and how to make healthy food choices. Here are some key principles of nutrition basics:

Macronutrients: Macronutrients are the three main types of nutrients that provide energy to your body: carbohydrates, proteins, and fats. Each macronutrient plays a different role in your body and has different effects on your weight and overall health. A balanced diet should include a mix of all three macronutrients.

Micronutrients: Micronutrients are vitamins and minerals that are essential for overall health and well-being. While they don't provide energy like macronutrients, they play a crucial role in maintaining healthy body function and preventing nutrient deficiencies.

Portion control: Portion control is an important aspect of healthy eating and weight loss. It's important to be mindful of portion sizes and avoid overeating. A general rule of thumb is to fill half of your plate with fruits and vegetables, one-quarter with lean protein, and one-quarter with whole grains or other complex carbohydrates.

Water intake: Staying hydrated is crucial for overall health and weight loss. Drinking water can help you feel fuller and more satisfied, which can help you eat less. Aim to drink at least eight glasses of water per day, or more if you're exercising or in a hot climate.

Mindful eating: Mindful eating involves paying attention to your body's hunger and fullness cues, and eating slowly and mindfully. This can help you avoid overeating and make healthier food choices.

Whole foods: Eating whole, unprocessed foods is an important part of a healthy diet. These

foods are typically higher in nutrients and fiber
than processed foods, and can help you feel
fuller and more satisfied.

By incorporating these nutrition basics into your
daily routine, you can make healthier food
choices, feel more satisfied and energized, and
achieve your weight loss goals over the
long-term.

**Understanding the role of nutrition in weight
loss**

Nutrition plays a critical role in weight loss. The
foods you eat provide your body with the energy
it needs to function, and the type and quantity of
food you consume can impact your weight loss
progress.

When it comes to weight loss, the goal is
typically to create a calorie deficit. This means
consuming fewer calories than your body burns
each day, which can help you lose weight over
time. However, it's important to note that not all
calories are created equal. The type and quality

of the foods you eat can have a significant impact on your weight loss progress.

One important aspect of nutrition for weight loss is macronutrient balance. As mentioned earlier, macronutrients are the three main types of nutrients that provide energy to your body: carbohydrates, proteins, and fats. Each macronutrient plays a different role in your body and can impact your weight loss progress in different ways.

For example, consuming too many carbohydrates, especially those that are high in refined sugars, can lead to spikes in blood sugar and insulin levels, which can contribute to weight gain. On the other hand, consuming too little protein can lead to muscle loss, which can slow down your metabolism and make it harder to lose weight.

In addition to macronutrient balance, it's important to pay attention to overall calorie intake. While creating a calorie deficit is necessary for weight loss, it's important to make sure that you're still consuming enough calories to support your body's basic needs and maintain muscle mass.

Another important aspect of nutrition for weight loss is food quality. Eating a diet that's high in whole, unprocessed foods can help you feel fuller and more satisfied, which can make it easier to stick to your weight loss goals. Additionally, these foods are typically higher in nutrients and fiber, which can help support overall health and weight loss.

Overall, understanding the role of nutrition in weight loss is crucial for achieving long-term success. By focusing on macronutrient balance, calorie intake, and food quality, you can make healthier food choices and create a sustainable, effective weight loss plan.

THE FUNDAMENTALS OF HEALTHY EATING

Healthy eating is a fundamental aspect of maintaining good health and achieving a healthy weight. Eating a balanced, nutrient-rich diet can provide your body with the energy and nutrients it needs to function properly and help you achieve your weight loss goals.

THE FUNDAMENTALS OF HEALTHY EATING INCLUDE:

Eating a variety of nutrient-dense foods: Nutrient-dense foods are those that are high in nutrients, such as vitamins, minerals, and fiber, but low in calories. Examples of nutrient-dense foods include fruits, vegetables, whole grains, lean proteins, and healthy fats.

Balancing macronutrients: As previously mentioned, macronutrients are the three main types of nutrients that provide energy to your body: carbohydrates, proteins, and fats. Eating a balanced diet that includes all three macronutrients can help you feel fuller for longer and provide your body with the nutrients it needs to function optimally.

Monitoring portion sizes: Eating too much of any food, even healthy foods, can lead to weight gain. Monitoring portion sizes can help you maintain a healthy calorie intake and support your weight loss goals.

Limiting processed and high-sugar foods: Processed foods are typically high in calories, unhealthy fats, and added sugars, which can contribute to weight gain and other health issues. Limiting processed and high-sugar foods can help you reduce your overall calorie intake and improve your overall health.

Staying hydrated: Drinking plenty of water and other hydrating fluids can help you feel fuller and reduce the likelihood of overeating. Additionally, staying hydrated can help support your body's natural detoxification processes and improve overall health.

Incorporating these fundamentals into your daily eating habits can help you achieve a healthier weight and improve overall health. By focusing on nutrient-dense foods, macronutrient balance, portion sizes, limiting processed and high-sugar foods, and staying hydrated, you can create a sustainable, effective approach to healthy eating and weight loss.

STRATEGIES FOR CREATING A SUSTAINABLE NUTRITION PLAN

Creating a sustainable nutrition plan is key to achieving long-term weight loss success. It involves finding a balance between healthy eating habits and realistic lifestyle factors. Here are some strategies for creating a sustainable nutrition plan:

Start with small changes: Rather than making drastic changes to your diet all at once, start by making small, gradual adjustments. For example, you could begin by adding more fruits and vegetables to your meals, or swapping out sugary drinks for water.

Set realistic goals: It's important to set realistic, achievable goals that fit into your lifestyle. For example, if you typically eat out several times a week, a goal to cook all of your meals at home may not be realistic. Instead, you could set a goal to cook at home three times a week and gradually increase from there.

Plan ahead: Planning your meals and snacks ahead of time can help you make healthier choices and avoid impulse decisions. Try prepping meals and snacks in advance, or keeping healthy options on hand for when hunger strikes.

Focus on balance: A balanced diet that includes a variety of nutrient-dense foods is key to sustainable weight loss. Aim to fill your plate with a combination of lean proteins, whole grains, fruits and vegetables, and healthy fats.

Practice mindful eating: Mindful eating involves paying attention to your body's hunger and

fullness cues and eating without distractions.
This can help you develop a better relationship
with food and avoid overeating.

Allow for flexibility: It's important to allow for
flexibility in your nutrition plan to avoid feeling
deprived or restricted. Incorporating occasional
treats or indulgences can help you stay on track
and prevent feelings of guilt or frustration.

Seek support: Having support from friends,
family, or a healthcare professional can help you
stay accountable and motivated on your weight
loss journey. Consider enlisting the help of a
registered dietitian or joining a support group for
added guidance and encouragement.

By implementing these strategies, you can create
a sustainable nutrition plan that supports your
weight loss goals and fits into your lifestyle.
Remember to be patient with yourself, as lasting
change takes time and effort. With consistency
and dedication, you can achieve your goals and
maintain a healthy weight for life.

INTRODUCTION TO EXERCISE AND MOVEMENT

Exercise and movement are essential components of a healthy lifestyle. They can improve physical health, mental well-being, and overall quality of life. Exercise refers to physical activity that is planned, structured, and repetitive for the purpose of improving or maintaining physical fitness, while movement encompasses any bodily activity, such as walking, bending, or lifting, that involves the contraction of muscles and the use of energy. Both exercise and movement can have numerous benefits, including reducing the risk of chronic diseases, improving cardiovascular health, strengthening muscles and bones, reducing stress and anxiety, and boosting cognitive function. With regular physical activity, individuals can experience improved energy levels, increased mobility, and a greater sense of overall wellness.

The benefits of exercise for weight loss

Exercise is a powerful tool for weight loss and can contribute significantly to achieving and maintaining a healthy weight. There are several benefits of exercise for weight loss, including:

Burning calories: When you exercise, you burn calories, which can lead to weight loss. The number of calories burned depends on the type of exercise, duration, and intensity. For example, a person who weighs 150 pounds can burn around 300 calories by jogging for 30 minutes.

Increasing metabolism: Regular exercise can increase your metabolism, which is the rate at which your body burns calories. A higher metabolism means your body will burn more calories even when you're at rest, which can lead to weight loss.

Building muscle: Exercise can help build lean muscle mass, which can increase your metabolic rate and help you burn more calories. Resistance training, such as weightlifting, is particularly effective at building muscle.

Reducing body fat: Exercise can reduce body fat, which is important for weight loss. Cardiovascular exercise, such as running or cycling, can be effective at reducing body fat.

Improving insulin sensitivity: Exercise can improve insulin sensitivity, which is important for weight loss. When your body is more sensitive to insulin, it can use glucose more efficiently, which can reduce the risk of weight gain and type 2 diabetes.

Enhancing mood: Exercise can enhance your mood and reduce stress and anxiety, which can help prevent emotional eating and promote healthy eating habits.

Overall, exercise is a key component of any weight loss plan. By incorporating regular physical activity into your lifestyle, you can burn calories, increase metabolism, build muscle, reduce body fat, improve insulin sensitivity, and enhance your mood, all of which can contribute to achieving and maintaining a healthy weight.

Types of exercise and finding what works for you
There are many different types of exercise, each with its unique benefits and challenges. Some of the most common types of exercise include:

Cardiovascular exercise: This type of exercise includes activities that raise your heart rate and get you breathing harder, such as running, cycling, swimming, or dancing. Cardiovascular exercise is great for improving cardiovascular health, burning calories, and boosting mood.

Resistance training: Resistance training involves using weights, resistance bands, or your own body weight to build strength and muscle. Resistance training is essential for maintaining strong bones and muscles, improving posture, and increasing metabolism.

Flexibility and stretching: Flexibility exercises, such as yoga or stretching, can help improve range of motion, reduce the risk of injury, and promote relaxation.

High-intensity interval training (HIIT): HIIT involves short bursts of intense activity, followed by periods of rest or lower-intensity exercise. HIIT can be an efficient way to burn calories, improve cardiovascular fitness, and build strength.

Finding the type of exercise that works for you can take some experimentation and trial-and-error. It's essential to consider your interests, fitness level, and any physical limitations you may have when choosing an exercise program. Some people prefer solo activities, such as running or swimming, while others enjoy group classes or team sports. It's also important to mix up your routine to prevent boredom and keep your body challenged.

If you're new to exercise or unsure where to start, consider working with a certified personal trainer or taking a fitness class. They can help assess your fitness level, develop a safe and effective exercise program, and provide guidance and motivation along the way.

In summary, there are many types of exercise, each with its unique benefits and challenges. Finding the type of exercise that works for you can take some experimentation, but with persistence and commitment, you can find a fitness routine that fits your lifestyle and helps you achieve your health and wellness goals.

Tips for staying motivated to exercise
Staying motivated to exercise can be challenging, especially when life gets busy or you don't see immediate results. However, there are several tips you can try to help you stay motivated and committed to your fitness routine:

Set realistic goals: Setting achievable goals can help you stay focused and motivated. Make sure your goals are specific, measurable, and realistic. For example, instead of setting a vague goal like "getting in shape," set a specific goal like "running a 5k in six months."

Find an exercise buddy: Exercising with a friend or family member can be a great way to stay motivated and accountable. Having someone to exercise with can make workouts more enjoyable and provide extra encouragement and support.

Mix up your routine: Doing the same workout every day can quickly become boring and demotivating. Try new exercises or activities to keep your routine fresh and challenging. You can also switch up the time of day or location where you exercise to add variety.

Reward yourself: Give yourself a reward for achieving your fitness goals or sticking to your routine. This can be anything from a new workout outfit to a massage or a favorite treat.

Keep track of your progress: Tracking your progress can help you stay motivated by showing you how far you've come. Keep a workout journal or use a fitness tracking app to monitor your progress and celebrate your achievements.

Focus on the benefits: Remind yourself of the benefits of exercise, such as improved health, increased energy, and reduced stress. Keeping these benefits in mind can help you stay motivated, even when you don't feel like working out.

Be kind to yourself: Finally, be kind to yourself and don't be too hard on yourself if you miss a workout or don't see immediate results. Remember that progress takes time, and every small step counts towards your overall fitness journey.

In summary, staying motivated to exercise can be challenging, but there are several tips you can try to help you stay committed to your fitness routine. Set realistic goals, find an exercise buddy, mix up your routine, reward yourself, track your progress, focus on the benefits, and be kind to yourself. With persistence and commitment, you can achieve your fitness goals and enjoy a healthier, happier life.

Mindful Eating and Portion Control

Mindful eating and portion control are two key strategies that can help individuals achieve a healthy and sustainable diet. Mindful eating involves paying attention to the present moment, and being aware of the sensory experience of eating. This means focusing on the taste, smell, texture, and appearance of food, as well as the physical sensations of hunger and fullness. Portion control, on the other hand, involves being mindful of the amount of food you eat, and choosing appropriate portion sizes to meet your nutritional needs without overeating.

Mindful eating can be practiced in a variety of ways. One approach is to eat slowly and mindfully, savoring each bite and taking time to appreciate the flavors and textures of the food. This can help you to become more aware of your hunger and fullness signals, and to avoid overeating. Another approach is to practice mindful food selection, by choosing foods that are nutrient-dense and satisfying, rather than simply relying on convenience or cravings.

Portion control can also be achieved through a variety of strategies. One approach is to use smaller plates, bowls, and utensils, which can help to reduce the amount of food you eat. Another strategy is to pre-portion your meals and snacks, by measuring out appropriate serving sizes ahead of time. This can help you to avoid mindlessly snacking or overeating.

Together, mindful eating and portion control can help individuals to develop a healthier relationship with food and achieve a sustainable, balanced diet. By practicing mindfulness and being aware of the amount and types of food you eat, you can achieve a more mindful, healthful approach to eating.

The importance of mindful eating in weight loss

Mindful eating is an essential component of successful weight loss. It involves being aware of the present moment, and fully engaging in the experience of eating. This means paying attention to the taste, texture, and smell of food, as well as the physical sensations of hunger and fullness.

One of the key benefits of mindful eating is that it can help individuals to tune in to their body's signals of hunger and fullness. By paying close attention to these cues, individuals can avoid overeating and reduce their overall calorie intake. Studies have shown that mindful eating can help individuals to eat less, without feeling deprived or hungry.

Another benefit of mindful eating is that it can help individuals to make healthier food choices. By being aware of the sensory experience of eating, individuals can choose foods that are satisfying and nutrient-dense, rather than simply relying on convenience or cravings. This can help individuals to achieve a more balanced and healthful diet.

Furthermore, mindful eating can help individuals to develop a more positive relationship with food. By approaching eating in a non-judgmental and compassionate way, individuals can reduce feelings of guilt or shame around food. This can help to reduce emotional eating, which is often a contributing factor to weight gain.

In summary, mindful eating is an important tool for weight loss. It can help individuals to tune in to their body's signals of hunger and fullness, make healthier food choices, and develop a more positive relationship with food. By incorporating mindful eating practices into their daily routine, individuals can achieve sustainable weight loss and long-term health benefits.

Strategies for practicing mindful eating and portion control

Practicing mindful eating and portion control are essential strategies for maintaining a healthy diet and achieving weight loss goals. Here are some effective strategies for incorporating mindful eating and portion control into your daily routine:

Pay attention to hunger and fullness cues: Before eating, take a moment to assess your hunger level. If you are feeling very hungry, it can be tempting to overeat or eat too quickly. On the other hand, if you are not feeling hungry, you may not need as much food as you think. During meals, pay attention to the physical sensations of fullness, and stop eating when you feel satisfied.

Use smaller plates and bowls: Using smaller plates and bowls can help to reduce the amount of food you consume. This is because smaller plates can make a serving of food appear larger, which can trick your brain into feeling more satisfied with less food.

Pre-portion your meals: Pre-portioning your meals can help you to eat the appropriate amount of food without overeating. Use measuring cups or a food scale to measure out the proper serving sizes for your meals and snacks.

Eat slowly and mindfully: Eating slowly and mindfully can help you to savor the flavors and textures of your food, and to become more aware of your hunger and fullness signals. Take time to chew your food thoroughly and put down your fork between bites.

Avoid distractions: Avoiding distractions while eating can help you to focus on your food and your body's signals. Turn off the TV, put down your phone, and try to eat in a calm and quiet environment.

Plan your meals ahead of time: Planning your meals ahead of time can help you to make healthier food choices and avoid mindless snacking or overeating. Take time each week to plan out your meals and snacks, and make a grocery list to ensure that you have healthy options on hand.

Incorporating these strategies into your daily routine can help you to develop a healthier relationship with food and achieve your weight loss goals. By practicing mindful eating and portion control, you can make lasting changes to your diet and improve your overall health and wellbeing.

Tips for incorporating mindful eating into your daily routine
Incorporating mindful eating into your daily routine can help you to develop a healthier relationship with food, reduce stress around eating, and improve your overall health and wellbeing. Here are some tips for incorporating mindful eating into your daily routine:

Slow down: Eating slowly and mindfully can help you to tune in to your body's hunger and fullness cues, and to savor the flavors and textures of your food. Take time to chew your food thoroughly and put down your fork between bites.

Eliminate distractions: Avoiding distractions while eating can help you to focus on your food and your body's signals. Turn off the TV, put down your phone, and try to eat in a calm and quiet environment.

Be present: Try to be fully present in the moment while eating, and avoid multitasking or thinking about other things. Focus on the sensory experience of eating, including the taste, smell, and texture of your food.

Listen to your body: Pay attention to your body's signals of hunger and fullness, and stop eating when you feel satisfied. Try to eat when you are hungry, rather than when you are bored or emotional.

Practice gratitude: Taking a moment to express gratitude for your food can help you to develop a more positive relationship with eating. Before eating, take a moment to give thanks for the nourishment that your food provides.

Choose nutrient-dense foods: Choosing nutrient-dense foods, such as fruits, vegetables, whole grains, and lean proteins, can help you to feel satisfied and nourished. Focus on eating a variety of colors and textures, and aim to include a balance of macronutrients in your meals.

Be patient and compassionate: Remember that developing a mindful eating practice takes time and patience. Don't be too hard on yourself if you slip up or make mistakes. Approach eating with a non-judgmental and compassionate attitude.

By incorporating these tips into your daily routine, you can develop a more mindful approach to eating and improve your overall health and wellbeing.

SECTION FOUR

OVERCOMING OBSTACLES

Obstacles are a natural part of life, and they can come in many different forms, whether it's a personal challenge, a setback at work, or a global crisis. Overcoming obstacles is an essential skill for success and personal growth. Here are some strategies for overcoming obstacles:

Reframe your mindset: The way you approach an obstacle can greatly impact your ability to overcome it. Instead of viewing obstacles as insurmountable challenges, try to reframe them as opportunities for growth and learning. This mindset shift can help you to stay motivated and focused.

Set goals: Setting clear and achievable goals can help you to stay on track and make progress towards overcoming your obstacles. Break your goals down into smaller, manageable steps and create a plan of action for how you will accomplish them.

Seek support: Don't be afraid to reach out to friends, family, or colleagues for support and encouragement. Talking to someone who understands what you are going through can be a valuable source of motivation and perspective.

Practice resilience: Resilience is the ability to bounce back from setbacks and adapt to change. Practicing resilience can help you to stay focused and positive in the face of obstacles. Try to stay flexible, adapt to new situations, and learn from your experiences.

Stay committed: Overcoming obstacles often requires persistence and dedication. Don't give up on your goals, even when things get difficult. Stay committed to your plan of action, and celebrate your progress along the way.

Learn from failure: Failure is a natural part of the process of overcoming obstacles. Instead of letting failure hold you back, try to learn from your mistakes and use them as an opportunity for growth and improvement.

Practice self-care: Overcoming obstacles can be emotionally and physically draining, so it's important to take care of yourself along the way. Practice self-care activities, such as exercise, meditation, or spending time with loved ones, to help manage stress and maintain a positive mindset.

By incorporating these strategies into your approach to overcoming obstacles, you can develop the resilience and determination needed to achieve your goals and overcome any challenge that comes your way. Remember to stay focused, seek support, and stay committed to your goals, and you will be well on your way to success.

Common obstacles to weight loss and how to overcome them

Losing weight can be a challenging process, and there are many obstacles that can make it difficult to achieve your goals. Here are some common obstacles to weight loss and strategies for overcoming them:

Lack of motivation: One of the most common obstacles to weight loss is a lack of motivation. To overcome this, it can be helpful to set clear and achievable goals, find a workout buddy or support group, or reward yourself for reaching milestones along the way.

Emotional eating: Emotional eating can derail weight loss efforts by causing you to consume more calories than you need. To overcome this, try to identify your triggers for emotional eating, such as stress or boredom, and find alternative ways to cope, such as going for a walk or practicing relaxation techniques.

Busy schedules: Busy schedules can make it challenging to find time to exercise or prepare healthy meals. To overcome this, try to schedule your workouts and meal prep in advance, or find ways to incorporate physical activity into your daily routine, such as taking the stairs instead of the elevator.

Plateaus: Weight loss plateaus can be frustrating and demotivating. To overcome this, try changing up your workout routine, increasing your intensity or duration, or focusing on making dietary changes, such as reducing your intake of processed foods or increasing your intake of fruits and vegetables.

Social pressure: Social pressure to indulge in unhealthy foods or skip workouts can be a significant obstacle to weight loss. To overcome this, try to communicate your goals and boundaries with your friends and family, find healthier alternatives for social activities, and surround yourself with supportive individuals.

Lack of knowledge: A lack of knowledge about healthy eating and exercise can make it challenging to achieve your weight loss goals.

To overcome this, educate yourself about healthy eating habits and exercise techniques, seek the guidance of a qualified professional, or find reliable sources of information online.

Medical conditions: Certain medical conditions, such as thyroid disorders or hormonal imbalances, can make it difficult to lose weight. To overcome this, seek medical advice from a qualified healthcare provider, and work with them to develop a customized plan that meets your unique needs.

By identifying these common obstacles to weight loss and using the strategies outlined above, you can develop a plan that works for you and overcome any challenges that come your way. Remember to stay focused on your goals, seek support

Strategies for dealing with setbacks and staying motivated

Setbacks are an inevitable part of life, and they can be frustrating and demotivating. However, it's important to remember that setbacks can also be valuable learning experiences, and they can help us build resilience and character. Here are some strategies for dealing with setbacks and staying motivated:

Reframe setbacks as opportunities: Rather than dwelling on the negative aspects of setbacks, try to view them as opportunities for growth and learning. Ask yourself what you can learn from the experience and how you can use that knowledge to improve in the future.

Set realistic goals: Setting goals that are achievable and realistic can help you stay motivated and avoid feeling overwhelmed by setbacks. Break larger goals down into smaller, manageable tasks, and celebrate each small accomplishment along the way.

Practice self-compassion: It's easy to be hard on ourselves when we experience setbacks, but practicing self-compassion can help us stay motivated and bounce back more quickly. Treat yourself with the same kindness and understanding that you would offer a good friend.

Seek support: Talking to a trusted friend, family member, or mentor can provide valuable perspective and support when you're feeling discouraged. They may be able to offer helpful advice or simply provide a listening ear.

Focus on what you can control: When setbacks occur, it's easy to feel powerless and overwhelmed. Instead, focus on what you can control and take action where you can. Even small steps can help you feel more empowered and motivated.

Stay positive: Cultivating a positive attitude can help you stay motivated and resilient in the face of setbacks. Practice gratitude, look for the silver lining in difficult situations, and focus on your strengths and accomplishments.

Take care of yourself: Self-care is crucial for maintaining motivation and resilience. Make sure to prioritize sleep, exercise, healthy eating, and other activities that help you feel energized and refreshed.

Remember, setbacks are a natural part of the learning and growth process. By adopting a positive mindset and utilizing these strategies, you can overcome setbacks and stay motivated to achieve your goals.

Building a support system for long-term success

Building a support system is an essential step for achieving long-term success in any area of life. Whether you're striving to achieve career goals, maintain a healthy lifestyle, or develop personal relationships, having a strong support network can provide you with the encouragement, accountability, and resources you need to stay motivated and achieve your goals.

Here are some steps you can take to build a support system for long-term success:

Identify your goals: To build an effective support system, you first need to know what you're working toward. Take the time to clarify your goals and the steps you need to take to achieve them.

Seek out like-minded individuals: Look for people who share your interests and goals, whether that's joining a professional organization or attending a local meetup group. Connect with individuals who are supportive and positive, and who are willing to offer encouragement and advice when needed.

Build strong relationships: Developing strong relationships with supportive individuals can help you stay motivated and accountable. Invest time and effort into building these relationships, and be willing to offer support in return.

Join a group or community: Joining a group or community that shares your interests can provide you with access to resources, knowledge, and support. Whether it's an online forum, a local club, or a support group, participating in a community can help you stay motivated and connected.

Seek professional support: Consider seeking the help of a coach, therapist, or other professional who can provide you with guidance and support as you work toward your goals. They can offer an objective perspective and help you overcome obstacles that may be holding you back.

Communicate your needs: Be open and honest with your support system about what you need from them, whether it's encouragement, accountability, or specific resources. Let them know how they can best support you, and be willing to reciprocate when they need support in return.

Remember, building a support system takes time and effort, but it can be a crucial step toward achieving long-term success. Surrounding yourself with positive, supportive individuals who share your goals and values can help you stay motivated, overcome challenges, and achieve your dreams.

CONCLUSION

Recap of the key principles of thinking big and working smart in your weight loss journey

When it comes to weight loss, thinking big and working smart are two important principles that can help you achieve long-term success. Here's a recap of the key principles involved:

Think big: Set ambitious, long-term goals that inspire and motivate you. Focus on what you want to achieve and why it's important to you. Break your goals down into smaller, achievable steps that you can work on each day.

Work smart: Develop a plan that takes into account your lifestyle, preferences, and habits. Make small changes to your diet and exercise routine that you can stick to long-term. Focus on building healthy habits that will support your weight loss goals.

Monitor progress: Keep track of your progress by regularly weighing yourself, taking measurements, and tracking your food and exercise. Use this information to adjust your plan as needed and stay motivated.

Stay accountable: Share your goals with others and seek out support from friends, family, or a weight loss group. Consider working with a coach or mentor who can provide guidance and accountability.

Practice self-care: Prioritize self-care by getting enough sleep, managing stress, and engaging in activities you enjoy. This can help you maintain your motivation and stay focused on your goals.

Celebrate success: Celebrate your achievements, no matter how small. This can help you stay motivated and remind you of your progress.

Remember, weight loss is a journey that requires patience, commitment, and perseverance. By thinking big and working smart, you can develop a plan that supports your goals and helps you achieve long-term success.

Tips for staying on track and reaching your goals

Staying on track and reaching your goals can be challenging, but with the right strategies and mindset, it is achievable. Here are some tips to help you stay on track and reach your goals:

Set clear and specific goals: Define your goals and make them as specific as possible. This will help you focus your efforts and measure your progress.

Break your goals into smaller, manageable steps: This will help you avoid feeling overwhelmed and make it easier to track your progress.

Create a plan: Develop a plan of action that outlines the steps you need to take to reach your goals. This will help you stay focused and on track.

Stay motivated: Stay motivated by reminding yourself why you are working toward your goals. Visualize yourself achieving your goals and how it will feel when you get there.

Track your progress: Keep track of your progress by measuring your results regularly. This will help you see how far you have come and keep you motivated.

Be accountable: Share your goals with others and seek support from friends, family, or a coach. This will help you stay accountable and motivated.

Stay positive: Focus on the positive and avoid negative self-talk. Celebrate your successes, no matter how small, and learn from your setbacks.

Stay flexible: Be open to adjusting your plan as needed. Life can be unpredictable, and it's important to be flexible and adapt to changes as they arise.

Take action: Take action every day, even if it's a small step. This will help you build momentum and move closer to your goals.

Practice self-care: Take care of yourself physically and emotionally by getting enough sleep, eating well, exercising regularly, and managing stress. This will help you stay focused and energized.

Remember, reaching your goals takes time, effort, and commitment. By staying on track, staying motivated, and staying accountable, you can achieve the success you desire.

Final thoughts on achieving lasting weight loss success.
Achieving lasting weight loss success is a journey that requires patience, commitment, and perseverance. While it can be challenging, it is achievable with the right mindset, strategies, and support system. Here are some final thoughts to keep in mind:

Focus on healthy habits: Rather than focusing solely on weight loss, focus on building healthy habits that you can sustain long-term. This includes eating a balanced diet, getting regular exercise, and practicing self-care.

Be patient: Losing weight takes time, and it's important to be patient with yourself. Don't get discouraged if you don't see results right away. Keep working at it, and you will see progress.

Stay motivated: Stay motivated by reminding yourself why you are working toward your goals. Focus on the benefits of a healthy lifestyle, and visualize yourself achieving your goals.

Stay accountable: Share your goals with others and seek out support from friends, family, or a weight loss group. Consider working with a coach or mentor who can provide guidance and accountability.

Practice self-compassion: Be kind to yourself and avoid negative self-talk. Celebrate your successes, no matter how small, and learn from your setbacks.

Stay flexible: Be open to adjusting your plan as needed. Life can be unpredictable, and it's important to be flexible and adapt to changes as they arise.

Celebrate success: Celebrate your achievements, no matter how small. This can help you stay motivated and remind you of your progress.

Remember, achieving lasting weight loss success is not just about reaching a certain number on the scale. It's about developing a healthy lifestyle that you can sustain long-term. By focusing on healthy habits, staying motivated, and staying accountable, you can achieve the success you desire.

Introduction:

It is well known that President Trump's and President Obama's supporters have strong opinions. It is therefore remarkable that it appears as of December 2019 no book has been written comparing their thoughts on various subjects in their own words. This is apparently the first. It is the author's hope that this collection of quotes will help illuminate their thinking on some of the most important topics of the day.

Chapter 1

Abortion Quotes